Leaders in Typhoid Fever

Leaders in Typhoid Fever

By

E. B. NASH, M.D.,

Author of
"Leaders in Homoeopathic Therapeutics."

GYAN

Published by

Gyan Publishing House
5, Ansari Road
Daryaganj, New Delhi-110002
Phone: 011-47034999, 9811692060
E-mail: books@gyanbooks.com

Distribution Network
gyanbooks.com
India, USA, Canada, UK, Australia, France

ISBN : 978-81-212-6599-7 (PB)
First Published, 1900

2nd Impression 2022

Printed at: Gyan Press, Delhi.

LEADERS IN TYPHOID FEVER
Author: E. B. NASH

Leaders

in

Typhoid Fever,

BY

E. B. NASH, M. D.,

Author of

" Leaders in Homœopathic Therapeutics."

1900.

DEDICATION.

To My Daughters,

Mary and Charlotte,

My Joy and Pride,

I Lovingly Dedicate

This Work.

PREFACE.

The profession have given such a welcome to "Leaders in Therapeutics" that I have been encouraged to write this present monograph. I have not given the description of the disease, but only the leading indications for the treatment, for the reason that it would only increase the price of the book, and be but a re-hash of what they already have in their libraries. Pathology is alike in all schools of medicine, but the homœopathic school is distinctive in its *treatment*. That is all that constitutes us a distinctive school of medicine. This is what we contend for, and claim for it superiority over all other known methods. I have attempted to improve upon our text-books by putting as nearly as possible the remedies together that naturally belong to the different forms and stages of this disease. It is my own experience through a period of nearly forty years. In my earlier practice I visited Adolph Lippe and asked him if he found the remedies that he recommended for typhoid hemorrhages twenty years before, as efficient now as then. He answered in his usual enthusiastic way: "I don't know. I don't have any cases of hemorrhage any more. I cure them." I was then astonished, but as I myself have come to know better how to use our remedies I understand him, for I have had but one case of hemorrhage in fifteen years, and aside from that one, not one that has run an unmitigated course. I am sure that under homœopathic treatment none will occur, and if they exceptionally do, we may blame ourselves and not our system. I hope finally by this, as well as my former work, to inspire especially our young men in the profession to a closer study of our superb homœopathic therapeutics, to the exclusion of all other fruitless hunts after something better.

E. B. NASH.

Cortland, N. Y.,
Oct. 12, 1899.

LEADERS IN TYPHOID FEVER.

LEADERS IN TYPHOID.

If there is any one disease which more than another cannot be prescribed for by name, it is this one. No disease is more varied in its symptoms during its inception, invasion, and course, and none more liable to spend its force in different localities in the subject. In one case the cerebral and nervous symptoms will greatly predominate so as to take the form of typhus cerebralis; in another, in the abdomen (Typhus abdominalis), and in still others, in the lungs and bronchi (Typhus pneumalis or Pneumo-typhus). Not only this, but during the course of any single case the form may change so as to assume these different manifestations. So in writing of the therapeutics of typhus we cannot arbitrarily divide the remedies into classes, but give the indications for their use in one or all forms according to symptomatic indications. Nevertheless there are certain remedies that are generally adapted to the first, second and third weeks, or stages, of the disease that it is well to recognize. To simply give a list of symptomatic indications beginning with *Aconite* and ending with *Zincum* is liable to be very confusing to the beginner, and he will have to take the time and have the experience to find out what the older practitioner might have told him at the start. We went over that route once and found it a "hard road to travel."

REMEDIES IN THE BEGINNING OF A CASE.

Every case must have its beginning, and if the symptoms during the *prodromic stage* are closely watched, and the homœopathic remedy properly applied, my word for it, very few cases need go on to a *course* of fever.

This is one place where the homœopathic treatment is superior to the old methods, for we may *treat the patient* before the disease may be certainly pronounced a confirmed case of typhoid or some such unwelcome diagnosis. I know we are sometimes charged with treating such cases and *claiming* to have "broken up" a fever, and it is not impossible that mistakes along that line have been made; but I submit that an old practitioner of abundant experience treating cases during a prevailing epidemic of the disease, would have to be given credit for knowing something of the case he was treating before it had reached the point where all the most serious diagnostic indications were developed, and be reasonably sure he had 'aborted" a case, which some, claim to be impossible. Those who claim to treat disease by name, with diagnosis fully established, must, to be consistent, wait until the time for preventing the disease is past. No wonder they claim that typhoid cannot be aborted. Such proceeding would be criminal with the homœopathist. In our indications for remedies we will follow out our own experience in the treatment of the disease, *prodroma* and all. Forty years ago if asked from our knowledge of remedies what were the remedies most likely to be needed in this (the prodromic) stage, we would have answered *Bryonia*, *Nux vomica*, *Rhus toxicod.*, *Pulsatilla* and *Belladonna*. It is different now, for there are two remedies that are oftener indicated than any of those named and which must be added, viz.: *Gelsemium* and *Baptisia*.

INDICATIONS FOR BRYONIA, GELSEMIUM AND BAPTISIA.

Of the three, *Bryonia*, *Gelsemium* and *Baptisia*, I cannot decide which is oftenest indicated in this stage. The symptoms which may be called "leaders" indicating *Bryonia* are: *Great lassitude or weakness. Pains in head, back and limbs, < on moving; white-coated tongue, dry parched lips and mouth, without or with thirst for water in large quantities at a time; loss of appetite, empty eructations and constipation; with restless sleep, which is accompanied by dreams of business, tiring him out, and particularly when the patient* *does not want to* **move,** *as all his bad feelings are* **greatly aggravated** *by it. One very characteristic symptom often but not always present is that the patient gets* **sick** *and* **faint** *when rising up from lying down.* Many cases begin with this array of symptoms, and my custom is to dissolve a few pellets of *Bryonia* 30th in two-thirds glass cold water and give dessert-spoonful doses once in two hours for three or four doses, and then wait for twenty-four hours. If there is amelioration at the end of that time I continue sac. lac. as long as improvement continues, and seldom have to repeat it or change the remedy. It cures, and that is the end of it.

Now the indications for *Gelsemium: Extreme muscular and nervous prostration*, with general **trembling** as a consequence. He wants to lie down, he feels *so weak*. If he attempts to walk the *legs tremble*, or the *hands tremble* if he attempts to lift them; the *tongue trembles* when he attempts to protrude it; the pulse becomes weak and slow, but is accelerated on the least motion; there is some chilliness, hands and feet cool, while there is *crimson flushing* of the face; inclination to drowsiness, or sleeps frequently, with incoherent muttering; head feels "big as a bushel," with vertigo and dimness of vision; tongue slightly coated, or not at all; speech thick, because the tongue, like all the rest of the muscles, "refuses to obey the will" from sheer inability, or from weakness, to do so. There is generally little or no thirst, no constipation or diarrhœa, and at this early stage, no stomach or bowel symptoms, unless it be, in some cases, the same sense of weakness (sometimes expressed as *goneness*) which is felt in general. *Drooping of the eyelids* is very characteristic and in keeping with the *general prostration.* Now this is the picture of a case which, if not helped out with *Gelsemium*, will surely go on to the lowest form of typhoid fever, and many are the cases that have been relieved and cured by me. Many patients have told me voluntarily that the effect of that medicine was wonderful. It sent a pleasureable thrill through their whole system and seemed to lift them right out of that prostration. This may seem to some like painting it too strongly, but having felt the same sensation in myself I cannot doubt it.

As to dose, I have received the same testimonial from the use of the 200th, 30th and the tincture, the latter two drops in the usual two-thirds glass cold water, dessert-spoonful doses. When the effect is apparent always stop the remedy and give sac. lac. as long as reaction continues.

Baptisia. Great prostration and soreness as if bruised in whatever position the patient lies; *the parts rested upon feel sore and bruised.*

(*Arnica.*) Stupor; falls asleep while being spoken to, or in the midst of his answer; face flushed, dusky, dark red, with a *stupid, besotted, drunken expression.* Tongue coated with a well-defined streak down the middle, at first white, but very soon turns brown, with red edges. Sometimes the tongue is large and flabby, with a red dry tip, but not distinctly triangular like *Rhus tox.* Exhalations and discharges early become *fetid, and offensive* breath, stool, urine and perspiration. *Nervous, cannot get to sleep because she cannot get herself together; feels scattered about, tosses around to get herself together.*

This is a picture of a rapidly advancing case of abdominal typhoid. The diarrhœa and decomposition of fluids set in early and progress rapidly, and if not speedily checked by *Baptisia* will come to the stage of *Arsenicum*, *Carbo veg.* or *Muriatic acid.* We could not do much with such cases, in the way of checking their progress, in their incipiency until Dr. Burt gave us *Baptisia*. Now we can, and have almost a sure relief in this remedy.

Again this remedy is like *Gelsemium*, efficacious in either the high, or low, preparations. The judgment of the prescriber must decide in each case. So far as my own experience in regard to dose is concerned, if I were obliged to discard all but one I would reserve the old Hahnemannian 30th potency; and I oftener prescribe it here than the higher or lower, and very seldom have to change. I think that mistakes are oftener made in the direction of too low, oft repeated, and long continued dosage than from the other extreme. The great majority of cases of typhus will in the beginning come within the range of these three remedies.

DIFFERENTIATIONS BETWEEN BRYONIA, GELSEMIUM AND BAPTISIA.

Then it is necessary that we understand them thoroughly, so as to apply them correctly, for a mistake at this stage is not easily corrected later, and may prove fatal. Let us compare a little. All three remedies have *muscular soreness* and *prostration;* but if the *soreness* is most prominent *Baptisia* leads; if the *prostration*, *Gelsemium*. *Gelsemium* and *Baptisia* are both drowsy with red face, but with *Baptisia* the mind is very clouded, with *Gelsemium* not nearly so much so. *Gelsemium* and *Bryonia* want to lie still, and dread motion—*Gelsemium* because he is *so weak*, *Bryonia* because his pains (especially in the head) are greatly aggravated. *Bryonia* is constipated, *Baptisia* diarrhœic, *Gelsemium* neither. With all three the face is red. *Baptisia* most so, "besotted," *Gelsemium* next. *Bryonia* least, and turns pale on rising or sitting up. Tendency to decomposition comes early with *Baptisia*, not so with the others. The delirium of *Bryonia* is about the business of the day, *Baptisia* cannot get himself together. *Gelsemium* not characteristic. The tongue of *Bryonia* is white, with *parched lips* and thirst. With *Gelsemium* the tongue is thinly coated or not at all, there is no thirst, and the tongue *trembles* when attempting to protrude it; while *Baptisia* is the only one that turns dark in a well defined streak through the middle in this stage. The urine with *Bryonia* is scanty and high colored, if changed at all, with *Gelsemium* may be profuse, and with *Baptisia* is scanty, dark and offensive. Other diagnostic differences between these remedies might be added, but enough is done to show that there is no reason for confusing them or difficulty in choosing between them.

NO ROUTINISM.

Now let no one, because I have taken pains to set forth the indications of these three remedies, so as to make them easily and quickly available, accuse me of a spirit of routinism; and let it not for a moment be supposed that I mean to convey that any other remedy indicated by the *symptoms* must be ignored, because there are other remedies that may in some individual case rule all these three out. For instance, if I should find a case in which the excessive soreness and bruised feeling, complaining of hardness of bed and prostration, and even coupled with a dark streak through the middle of the tongue, so strongly indicating *Baptisia* as above described, and the history of the case should show that the patient had come to this state through the strain of overwork and fatigue, I should consider and compare *Arnica*, notwithstanding this remedy is not generally useful until later in the course of ordinary fevers. *Rhus toxicodendron* also will come strongly to mind in cases arising from similar causes.

In other cases in which those who, during an epidemic of fevers, had come down after a long strain of night watching and broken rest in taking care of the sick, no remedy so helps them as *Cocculus; Cuprum stands* next.

PULSATILLA AND NUX VOMICA.

Pulsatilla. If there is *much chilliness* yet the patient cannot bear to be in a *close room*, it oppresses her; *white tongue without thirst;* bad taste in the mouth; sour eructation, and especially if the *menses retard*, or are suppressed; very greatly discouraged, or gloomy and lachrymose.

Nux vomica. In the case of sedentary men who come down with severe headache and constipation, with frequent desire for stools, which do not satisfy, or ineffectual efforts at stool, and especially if with very *high fever and bright red face there is constant desire to be covered, for he is chilly if he moves or is uncovered in the least.* The patient is very nervous, sensitive and easily affected by external impressions.

I put these two remedies here together because I think they belong here. The *Nux vomica* picture is predominently found among men; the *Pulsatilla* in women. If some should object that these are not typhoid fever remedies, because they do not create or cause the pathological changes that characterize a fully developed case of this disease, I answer that any remedy having the symptoms of the *patient*, even though they be only subjective symptoms, is homœopathic to the case, and that if applied when and where it belongs the pathological changes so characteristic may be *averted.* *To meet and defeat in this way disease at the very outset is one of the chief excellencies of our art as compared with the old school of medicine.* The "practice of medicine made easy" by prescribing the one remedy for all cases of one (nominal) disease, without regard to the individual, or peculiar, symptoms in the case, is simply in the line of the old mistake of *Quinine* for malarious affections, *Mercury* for syphilis, etc., etc. We know the result.

It is not possible to tell what exceptional remedy will be the indicated one in the first, or, indeed, in any stage of typhoid fever.

REMEDIES FOLLOWING THE FIRST OR PRODROMAL STAGE OF TYPHOID FEVER.

Now we will take up the remedies as they are most frequently indicated after the stage of invasion is established, in case we are not able to "abort." Sometimes with our best efforts we are not able to "abort" the case. And in some cases we are called in too late to do so. Nevertheless, we need not despair of so modifying the disease during the first and second weeks so as to render the case a mild one, and in most instances to entirely avert the stage of ulceration and hemorrhage, which is always serious and sometimes fatal. *Baptisia*, *Bryonia*, *Lachesis*, *Phosphoric acid*, *Rhus toxicodendron* and, exceptionally, *Gelsemium* should here hold first place.

BAPTISIA AND GELSEMIUM.

I have seen the whole aspect of a very serious case changed to a favorable one on the ninth or tenth day by *Baptisia* 30th, being guided to its selection by its characteristic mind symptom, and the same with *Gelsemium* 200th after *Bryonia* had done all it could, the guiding symptom being the **trembling** so characteristic of this drug. So it would be a great mistake to lose sight of these remedies, because as a general thing they are most useful in the beginning.

BRYONIA.

Bryonia more than either of these is liable to be *the remedy* all through the case. As long as the white or, may be, yellowish tongue, parched lips and thirst, constipation, pain in the head and delirium in mild forms *about the business of the day* and *dread of motion* continues *Bryonia* must be continued.

RHUS TOXICODENDRON.

But if, as is often the case, diarrhœa supervenes, the tongue becomes *dry as a board* and especially if *red at the tip in the shape of a triangle;* pointing backward;

again, if the delirium and stupor increase with low form of muttering much of the time, and the patient *cannot lie still* but must *toss and change position* every little while, as if temporarily relieved of suffering by so doing, *Bryonia* is no longer "in it," but *Rhus toxicodendron*, and no two remedies follow each other better than these.

Of course other symptoms will often be present, but these are reliable " leaders " and no case needs *Rhus toxicodendron* without them.

PHOSPHORIC ACID.

But the case may not take on this *restless* form, but while a *stupid, indifferent or apathetic condition* remains the patient lies on his back very still. He doesn't want to talk and answers slowly; the whole case seems one of *torpor.* In addition to this, there is diarrhœa, actual or threatened, with *excessive meteoric distension of the abdomen*, with great rumbling and noise as from water; if diarrhœa, it is painless, yellow, watery, or very *light colored*, even WHITE. For this condition there is no remedy like *Phosphoric acid.* I have oftener found it indicated in men, young, or married, whom I suspected, or knew, had been to excess in onanism or venery.

ARNICA.

Arnica has an apathetic condition, or indifference, similar to *Phosphoric acid*, but the *Arnica* depression is more profound as is also that of *Baptisia*, for they both *go to sleep in the midst of answering a question.* The stupor-apathy overpowers them, but here the similarity ends.

LACHESIS.

Lachesis is one of our best remedies in typhoid, and may be indicated in any except the first and last stages. Its symptomatic indications are very positive and reliable, as follows: Muttering stupor, even almost complete insensibility; sleeps with mouth open; dry, red, or black tongue, which, on attempting to protrude, *trembles and catches on the lower teeth* (this indicates great weakness). The stools are *very offen-*

sive, whether formed or not, and if there is hemorrhage, it is of dark decomposed blood, with sometimes an appearance as of flakes of *charred straw* in it; the throat seems full, with loud breathing, and the patient, though stupid, is very restless, seems to feel suffocated and does not *like to have anything about the throat or chest*, throws off the covers therefrom; but, as is not the case with other remedies, if he does get any real sleep all his sufferings are *greatly aggravated.* The more he sleeps the *worse he feels.* This cannot be emphasized too strongly. I have seen several just such cases as this and can testify that *Lachesis* is a "friend indeed." Time and again I have seen a serious case changed to a mild and easily managed one, within twenty-four hours, by the 200th potency of this wonderful remedy.

I will, I hope, be pardoned if I seem enthusiastic here, for it is hard to withhold my praise justly due such an old and faithful servant. It is sometimes a little difficult to choose between this and some other remedies having equally depressing effects upon the sensorium, but if we do not allow ourselves to be *hurried* in the examination of such serious cases, but take time, examine closely, and choose deliberately, it will *pay*.

WHEN APPARENTLY WELL CHOSEN REMEDIES DO NOT ACT.

The elder Lippe once said to me that *Lachesis* was a remedy that could, like *Sulphur*, sometimes be used on the indication, "when other apparently well-chosen remedies do not act." I have found this true to this extent even as I have with *Sulphur*. When between *Rhus tox.* and *Arsenicum*, or *Hyoscyamus* and *Opium*, where the depression and stupor or weakness had points of resemblance, or one or the other of them had been tried, or the case was not developed in *all* the characteristics of one remedy, that a few doses of *Lachesis* did seem to develop and clear up the case so as to make the indications more unmistakable. But I believe it must be true that if all the symptoms had come out at that time *Lachesis* must have been the indicated remedy, for there are no exceptions to *similia similibus curantur*. It is seldom that we find a case of typhoid fever that can be carried through the course on one remedy. If, however, the exact similimum is prescribed at the beginning there will be no running through a course. If we are not reasonably sure of our remedy, on account of an undeveloped case, it is better to wait a while than to "fire in the dark," for we are liable to do more harm than good. To be sure it sometimes takes more courage to stand than to fight, but we want to know what we are fighting and where to aim our guns.

ARSENICUM ALBUM.

The remedy that is very likely to be necessary if the case goes on from bad to worse, notwithstanding the use of one or more of those already noticed, is *Arsenicum album.* I know that some who are considered authority have taught that *Arsenicum* throughout its pathogenesis more closely resembles in all its stages a genuine typhoid than any other, and, therefore, that it is good practice to give it from the beginning, and all through, without much regard to differentiation between it and other remedies, except it be to drop in (interpolate) for particular symptoms some other remedy in alternation for the purpose of quieting those symptoms, while *Arsenicum* keeps getting in its work in a *general* way.

Acting on such authority, I inclined in my earlier practice to that way. But I found after a while that cases treated thus would oftener run the whole course than otherwise; first, because many cases did not need *Arsenicum* at all, and of course were not benefited; next, because even in the cases where it was the remedy the continued dosing that I did with it hindered re-action, sometimes, I fear, greatly damaging, if not *killing*, my patient, with the remedy which, properly used, might have cured him.

I saw such a case in consultation with a Jersey City physician, who was *holding his patient down* with *Arsenicum* 3d in oft repeated doses, with an occasional dose of *Mercurius corrosivus* 3d for the particular symptoms of *tenesmus.* That patient, a strong young man, after a very long sickness, recovered, I *think*, in spite of bad treatment. I know there is a better way, for I have tried both and proven it to my satisfaction.

I will not here undertake to give all the symptoms set down in the text-books that may be found present in an *Arsenicum* case, but rather what I have found to be the "Leading" ones—where the powers of life seem to be greatly exhausted; great *restlessness* and *anxiety*, which is manifested by constantly moving head and limbs, while trunk lies still on account of too great weakness; tongue either red, dry, cracked, or black and stiff; *excessive thirst* for little at a time; *burning* in stomach or bowels, or both; meteoristic distension of the abdomen; diarrhœa watery, brownish, or bloody and *offensive; all worse at midnight, especially about one o'clock.* Here are only a few symptoms, but every *Arsenicum* case has them, or a good share of them, sure. The prostration is very great, and so is that of *Carbo veg.* and *Muriatic acid*, but in neither of these two is the prostration accompanied by the excessive *anguish* and *restlessness* of *Arsenicum*. They have gotten past that. The thirst of *Arsenicum* is no greater than that of *Bryonia*, but *Bryonia* wants large quantities at long intervals, while *Arsenicum* cannot take large quantities at a time, for it distresses and nauseates, or causes vomiting. The excessive restlessness occurs equally under *Arsenicum* and *Rhus toxicodendron*, but there is not the same degree of *prostration* with *Rhus toxicodendron*. The patient can, and does, turn, or throw, himself from side to side, and seems to be temporarily *relieved* thereby, while if the *Ar-*

senicum patient makes out to move himself he is *greatly exhausted* and *made worse.*

The general aggravation of *Rhus toxicodendron* is also during the latter part of the night, but not so characteristically at one o'clock. I think that of all the remedies we have so far considered, *Rhus tox.* and *Arsenicum* come nearest together, and I have found very few cases of typhoid where after *Rhus tox.* had done all it could (unless it cured the case which it sometimes does), *Arsenicum* was not the next remedy.

Now, with *Arsenicum*, as, indeed, with any other remedy, the earlier positive indication for its use is recognized, the better the effect following its administration, either to cure at once or at least to so greatly modify the case as to render the further conduct of it comparatively easy.

CARBO VEGETABILIS AND MURIATIC ACID.

After *Arsenicum* has done all it can, if the case goes on from bad to worse, we have still two remedies that offer hope. They are *Carbo vegetabilis* and *Muriatic acid.*

Carbo veg. can sometimes save life after all else fails. It is the stage of collapse, dissolution of the blood, and paralytic conditions beyond the reach of anything else. There is almost total obliviousness to everything. The face is *deathly pale*, sunken, hippocratic, cold. There may be hemorrhages from nose, mouth or anus, one or all at a time, and always with that *deathly paleness.* Abdomen meteoristic, with rumbling and gurgling of wind. Diarrhœa of cadaverous smell and often involuntary. Rattling breathing in bronchi, filled with mucus (threatened paralysis of lungs). The circulation becomes so weak that the blood *stagnates in the capillaries*, with cyanotic blueness of face, lips and tongue. The nose and breath grow cold, as do also the *extremities* which are covered with cold sweat, and under the extremely weak heart action the breathing becomes so difficult that the patient from *hunger for oxygen*, gasps, "fan me!

fan me!" All this indicates beginning paralysis of the heart (heart failure) and is a picture of complete torpor of the vital forces. The prostration is beyond that of *Arsenicum* even, which is always more or less associated with erethism. I have seen such a case revive and completely recover under the action of *Carbo veg.*, and let me mention right here that if the improvement brought about by *Carbo veg.* in such a case needs further help, *China officinalis* is generally the best remedy. No two remedies that I know of, oftener complement each other better.

Muriatic acid is another remedy that almost vies with *Carbo veg.* in these almost hopeless cases of typhoid. The vital depression is very great. *Febris stupida.* The weakness is so great that the patient constantly sinks or *slides down in the bed*, with loud moaning and groaning during sleep. Muttering and unconsciousness even when awake; lower jaw dropped; tongue *shrunken* (sometimes to a third its natural size) and dry, like leather, patient cannot move it at will even when conscious; putridity; involuntary stools while passing urine; bleeding from the anus; pulse intermitting every third beat. In one of these desperate cases that I cured with this remedy the tongue and gums were covered with deep bluish ulcers, otherwise the characteristic symptoms above named were present, especially the *sliding down* in bed, *paralyzed tongue* and *involuntary bloody stools* and *urine.*

It is always a source of comfort to the physician, when conducting a case of typhoid, to feel that he has two such remedies as *Carbo veg.* and *Muriatic acid* in reserve, even tho' it is true that very few cases well managed ever need them.

OPIUM AND NUX MOSCHATA.

Perhaps here is as good a place as any to introduce two remedies that are especially adapted to those cases that come under the head of *febris stupida*, viz., *Opium* and *Nux moschata.* *Opium* here leads all the remedies. The *stupor is com-*

plete; almost impossible to rouse him; lies speechless sometimes, with open or half-open eyes; face *dark red* and *bloated; stertorous breathing;* involuntary stools and retained urine. This state may alternate with wild delirium with loud talking, laughing or singing and attempts to escape, but the leading indications are those pertaining to the *stupid state.* On account of this alternation of stupor and wild delirium it may sometimes be difficult to choose between *Opium* and *Hyoscyamus*, which has the same, but close comparison will generally decide.

Nux moschata, which I have introduced alongside *Opium*, is not after all so near it as *Hyoscyamus*, but is nevertheless one of our remedies for *febris stupida*. It seems to me that it comes closer to *Phosphoric acid* in its symptomatology than any other remedy, though the stupor is greater. As I wrote in my *Leaders in Homœopathic Therapeutics*, page 277: "The effect upon the brain, while producing a sleepiness and dullness almost equal to *Opium*, is of an entirely different character, the *Opium* being seemingly due to fullness of the blood vessels and pressure (evidenced by the bloated red face and injected eyes), while that of *Nux moschata* seems to be a benumbing of the very nerve substance itself. Notwithstanding both *Opium* and *Nux moschata*, on account of the stupor, are frequently indicated in typhoid, the choice between them is not difficult. The leading symptoms as recorded by *Raue* and in parenthesis accredited to (Hering confirmed by Nash) are: —

Profound coma.

Lying silent, immovable, insensible.

Difficult comprehension, slowness of ideas.

Dwells long on her answer, or does not answer at all.

Very deaf.

Putrid colliquative diarrhœa.

Rolling, rumbling and gurgling of the bowels.

Dreamy state, with drowsiness and falling of the eyelids, *dryness of tongue, mouth and throat*, with fullness of stomach and loss of appetite.

In the evening the dryness is so great that the tongue sticks to the roof of the mouth. *Yet there is no thirst.*"

I have quoted this entire from Raue. A comparison of this remedy with *Phosphoric acid* will show how closely they resemble each other.

Quoting again from *Leaders*, page 278: "I once had a case of typhoid fever of the *nervosa stupida* variety. On account of the stupor the yellow, watery diarrhœa, and rumbling and bloating of the abdomen, I thought surely *Phosphoric acid* must help; but it did not. I finally discovered the *excessive dryness of the mouth*, which had escaped my attention before. This completed the picture for *Nux moschata.* Under the action of the 200th potency the patient rapidly improved unto complete recovery.

So we must "watch out" when the *seemingly* indicated remedy does not cure, for it may not be *Sulphur*, *Opium*, *Laurocerasus* or *Psorinum* that will have to be given, as we said when writing upon *Opium* and *Sulphur;* but we have not, no matter what the "seemings," chosen the homœopathic remedy at all, and as in this case some symptom may appear that will change the prescription entirely. "*Nux moschata* is not so well understood or often used as it should be."

REMEDIES FOR PNEUMO-TYPHUS, PHOSPHORUS, HYOSCYAMUS, RHUS TOX. AND SULPHUR.

For *Pneumo-typhus* the leading remedies are *Phosphorus*, *Hyoscyamus*, *Rhus toxicod.* and *Sulphur.* We have occasionally a case in which the typhoid poison "seems to localize principally in the chest, causing hypostasis of the lungs, pneumonia or violent bronchitis, while the characteristic affections of the small intestines are comparatively light, or even wanting." Such conditions used to be called *complications.* In such a case, if there is *hard dry* cough (*Bryonia*) with tightness of the chest, or the cough is more loose with rusty expectoration, cough worse in the *evening until midnight*, and especially worse lying on the *left side* there may be hepatization, especially of the *lower right lung*, these symptoms being so prominent as to cover to quite a degree the other typhoid symptoms, *Phosphorus* may be given, and may, with the relief of these symptoms, change the whole case favorably and usher the patient into the road that leads to recovery. In such a case it is quite common to find a serious degree of *cardiac weakness*, for which *Phosphorus* is also one of our best remedies.

While this remedy has not the strongly-developed characteristics in this disease that many others have, it has, on the other hand, a general wide range of action that lets it in on what Jahr used to call "*tout ensemble*" of the symptoms. The indications for *Rhus tox.* in these cases are already given, except the pneumonic infiltration, which must be added. *Phosphorus* is hardly ever indicated, though it may be, before *Rhus tox.*, but follows it well if the latter remedy cannot control the pneumonic manifestations.

Sulphur is a very important remedy here, especially in subjects having a psoric history, and if given as soon as the lung trouble begins to develop, and, especially, at the beginning of the process of lung infiltration, recognized by the crepitation sound, may render the use of *Phosphorus* unnecessary. If, however, we have not given the *Sulphur* at this stage, and hepatization has occurred, the time when red hepatization is completed and the third, or gray stage is beginning, is just the time when *Phosphorus* can do its *best work.* It performs miracles here, as I have often witnessed in both pneumonia and pneumo-typhus.

A few of the most characteristic indications in addition to those already given are:

Bright red lips.

Redness of edges and tip of tongue.

Diarrhœa < *early in the morning, with great prostration after stool.*

Flushes of high fever followed by prostration.

BURNING OF FEET, will stick them out of bed even when unconscious.

There is no doubt of the utility of *Sulphur* here, and if it does not absolutely introduce the stage of convalescence, will often so modify the case that other remedies can easily conduct it to a favorable *finis*.

In regard to *Hyoscyamus* in these cases, I have learned to regard it very highly. I cannot see that it makes any difference whether we are treating a case of typhoid-pneumonia or pneumo-typhus if we have the symptomatic indications present. Typhus simply means, literally, *smoke*, *stupefaction*, that is all, and in either of these diseases *Hyoscyamus* smokes, or stupefies more than *Phosphorus* or *Rhus toxicodendron*, and that is one indication for its preference in such cases. Otherwise we will try to give the indications for *Hyoscyamus* more fully when we treat *Belladonna* and *Stramonium*, the other two of the trio of delirious remedies.

ARNICA MONTANA.

Before doing this I want to call attention to *Arnica montana*, a remedy that has other important uses than those arising from traumatic causes. The reason why *Arnica* is such a regal remedy for the effects of injuries, especially bruises, is because in the provings it produces soreness and a sensation as if bruised. Now if these same sensations occur in disease, even without the traumatic element, *Arnica* should still be the homœopathic remedy. And so it is, for the first and most important symptom indicating it in fevers is the *sore and bruised sensation* that makes the patient want to continually move or be moved, because he cannot lie on the sore parts; he complains that *the bed is too hard. Baptisia* comes nearest to *Arnica* in this symptom. This is different from *Rhus tox.*, for then the patient must move because the muscles *ache* and are temporarily relieved by motion. *Arnica* is:

Weary, *weak* and **stupid.**

Complains of no particular pain, only the *sore*, *bruised* sensation.

Sits, or lies, as if stupid, forgets the word he is speaking.

Bleeds from the nose.

Face may be *red and hot*, *while the rest of the body is cool* (*Phytolacca*).

Unnoticed micturition and *defecation.*

Brown streak through the middle of the tongue (*Baptisia*).

Suggillations under the skin.

Foul smelling breath.

Distension of the abdomen.

Brown or white diarrhœa.

A study of *Arnica* shows strong similarity between it and *Baptisia*, so far as symptoms go, but I have found as a rule that the *Arnica* is oftener useful later rather than in the beginning of typhoids. It is sometimes lost sight of in the popular teaching that it is only to be used in cases connected with *trauma.*

CEREBRAL TYPHUS AND ITS REMEDIES.

Now we come to a very important part of our subject, the treatment of cerebral typhus. The leading remedies here are: *Belladonna*, *Hyoscyamus*, *Stramonium*, *Apis mellifica*, *Helleborus niger* and *Zincum metallicum*.

The first three have wild delirium so nearly alike that if this were all it would not always be an easy task to choose between them, but happily aside from this there are symptoms peculiar to each, and again even in those that are similar there are different degrees of intensity; for instance—*Hyoscyamus* has greater *stupor* than either of the others, when there is stupor.

Belladonna has more active congestion to the brain, with drowsiness and inability to go to sleep, or on the verge of falling off into, or if he does fall asleep, *starts and jumps* as if frightened, there is red face and eyes and *throbbing* of the carotids, the skin is very hot, which *under the bed clothes* may be found *moist* or *sweating*, i. e., *covered parts sweat.* I give these as characteristics for this remedy, and they do not occur, or at least to anything like the same degree, under the other two remedies.

Belladonna is most apt to be

useful in the beginning of tumultuous cases, exceptionally later.

Hyoscyamus, oftener indicated in true typhoid than either of the three, has, aside from the wild delirium—

Entire loss of consciousness, and of the functions of the organs of sense.

The delirium continues while awake; sees persons who are not and have not been present, muttering, with *picking of the bed clothes ;* staring at surrounding objects; reaching into the empty air for them.

Comprehends slowly, if at all, and stares at the physician.

Tongue red, dry, brown, cracked

or paralyzed; puts it out slowly if requested, and forgets to draw it back, or cannot put it out at all.

Sordes on teeth and cadaverous smell from the mouth.

Urine retained, suppressed or involuntary.

Paralysis of sphincter ani and vesica; stools and urine unnoticed (*Arnica*).

Twitching of muscles, *subsultus tendinum.*

Sleeplessness with staring eyes; or constant sleep with muttering.

Roseola spots on chest and abdomen.

This is a picture of *Hyoscyamus*, and whatever the general remedy may be during the *course* of the fever it is here indispensable.

ALTERNATION.

Hahnemann alternated *Bryonia* and *Rhus tox.* in a certain epidemic, not giving one one hour and the other the next, as is the manner of bunglers, but when indicated by the symptoms from day to day using the one remedy alone until the effects were visible. I shall have, further on, occasion to relate two cases in which I was obliged to do the same.

I mention this here because I wish to say (without the possibility of being charged with the heresy of alternation or rotation of remedies) that I have observed cases in which such alternation of *Hyoscyamus* and *Rhus tox.* was, I believe, entirely in accord with our law of cure, and, again, that the cases that are best covered by *Rhus tox.* in their generality are just the ones in which *Hyoscyamus* is most likely to be needed by way of interpolation.

I have already spoken of this remedy in its bearing upon pneumo-typhus, where it is invaluable. I do not think that with these symptoms so plainly given, we need give *Belladonna* or *Stramonium* by mistake.

STRAMONIUM.

Stramonium delirium differs from that of the other two remedies in the degree of its *intensity*.

The raving is something awful. Singing, laughing, grinning; whistling; screaming, praying piteously or swearing hideously, and above all remedies **loquacious.** Again the patient throws himself into all shapes corresponding to his changeable delirium, crosswise, lengthwise, rolled up like a ball, or stiffened out by turns, or *especially* repeatedly *jerks up suddenly his head* from the pillow. Things look crooked or oblique to him.

The whole inner mouth as if raw; the tongue after a while may become stiff or paralyzed. Stools loose, blackish, smelling like carrion, or no stool or urine. Later there may be complete loss of sight, hearing, and speech with dilated, immovable pupils and drenching sweat which brings no relief, and death must soon close the scene unless *Stramonium* helps them out.

By way of still further comparison *Stramonium* is the most wildly loquacious.

Hyoscyamus is the most insensibly STUPID.

Belladonna in this respect stands half way between.

Stramonium, throws himself about, jerking head from pillow.

Hyoscyamus, twitches, picks and reaches, otherwise lying pretty still.

Belladonna, starts or jumps when falling into or awaking from sleep.

All have times of *wanting to escape*.

APIS MELLIFICA, HELLEBORUS NIGER AND ZINCUM METALLICUM IN BRAIN TYPHUS.

With this rendering of this superb trio we must leave it to the practitioner to make his own further differential diagnosis, fully aware that we have not by any means exhausted the subject, and go on to consider the remaining three of our leading remedies for brain typhus, viz.: *Apis mellifica*, *Helleborus niger* and *Zincum metallicum*.

Apis mellifica has again and again rendered me such good service in advanced cases of cerebral typhus that I have learned to prize it very highly. Aside from anything laid down in the text-books in connection with this disease, I place apathy, or *stupor*, interrupted with occasional *sharp screams*, first and have frequently found it useful; or this may alternate with long continued spells of *whining*. Another characteristic is *general trembling*. This trembling is continuous and violent; shakes the bed; hands have to be held they tremble so. It comes late in the course of the disease, like the trembling of *Zincum metallicum*.

This is different from *Gelsemium*, which comes early and is aggravated on motion, or does not show unless they undertake to move or do something with the hands, or feet. My attention was first called to this *whining and trembling* of *Apis mel.* by a case cured by Dr. Ad. Lippe in one of the first volumes of the "*Hahnemannian Monthly*," and afterwards vouched for by the doctor himself by word of mouth; and as I have verified it several times since, myself, I think it is very reliable. In addition to this the abdomen may be distended, sore and very *sensitive to touch*, with foul, bloody, or involuntary stools, the anus sometimes remaining open (*Phosphorus*); or on the contrary the abdomen may be sunken, even hollowed out like a boat, with no stool, and very scanty or suppressed urine. In either case the patient is very weak, sliding down in bed (*Mur. acid*), and the skin alternately *hot and dry*, or *profusely sweating*. I promised a little way back to give a case in which I found it necessary to alternate as Hahnemann did *Bryonia* and *Rhus toxicodendron*—two remedies.

CLINICAL CASES.

Case. A boy 12 years of age (in a family in which one had already died of hemorrhage of the bowels and another lay sick of the same disease in the abdominal form) was taken with typhoid fever and grew steadily worse until the third week, when the following symptoms were present:

Complete stupor; entire unconsciousness; pupils greatly dilated, with no reaction to light; and hearing gone. All this interrupted by occasional piercing screams; abdomen so sunken and empty that the vertebral column could be felt through its walls; no stool for two weeks and for forty-eight hours at one time not a drop of urine. He would lie for a day or so in this stupor, then would involuntarily begin to jerk his head forward up from the pillow, and with a yell carry it around in a sort of semi-circle and drop it back again, continually trying to talk, which he could not do on account of the stiff or paralyzed condition of the tongue; then again would lapse into the stupor with screams. *Apis mellifica* alone did not control the whole condition, so I gave the *Stramonium*, when, with the jerking of the head, and loquacious delirium was on, and between the two remedies he began to improve, the paroxysms becoming shorter and more mild, then ceasing entirely. The urine became abundant, and the boy began to notice his attendants. The first word he spoke ten days after he became conscious was "*maw!*" (calling his mother), the next "pawidge" (porridge). His diet had been oat meal porridge all through the course.

Two other cases essentially the same, one a school teacher, the other the wife of the professor of mathematics in our State Normal School, were treated the same way and made perfect recoveries. The late lamented Dr. H. V. Miller, one of the best prescribers I ever knew, saw the last one in consultation with me and pronounced a decidedly unfavorable prognosis, but was surprised and delighted at the outcome. I have also prescribed it alone in cases which had the stupor with screaming without the alternate condition described above with equally good results. In almost all cases of the *Apis* kind look for an increase of urine before the other symptoms improve.

APIS AND SULPHUR.

One thing I wish to mention here, viz., that if in such a case *Apis mellifica* did not act promptly an intercurrent dose of *Sulphur* often seemed to help it. There must have been psora in such a case, and I know that the two remedies follow each other beautifully when indicated by the symptoms. Now, for fear that some one may accuse me of teaching alternation or rotation of remedies, as is the practice of too many in our school, let me say that the cases which call for even such alternation as was necessary here, are very rare, and you will distinctly remember that this was not the hourly or two hourly rotation practiced by such.

Such alternation and rotation is neither necessary nor scientific. No good prescriber will do it.

A CLINICAL CASE ILLUSTRATING THE USE OF HELLEBORUS NIGER.

Helleborus niger is another remedy which, though not often indicated in typhoid, is sometimes, and nothing can take its place. To illustrate its sphere I will give another case from practice.

This was another boy about twelve or fourteen years of age. After two weeks of a very severe run of the fever, the whole force of the disease seemed to concentrate in the brain. The loose stools stopped, and the urine, too, and he lay dead to all signs of consciousness; the eyes remained wide open and still; shoving a bright lamp right up to them made no impression upon the widely dilated pupils. He looked *idiotic*, and the heart beat was weak and very slow, "only the brain seems to be the invaded part of the body."

Under the action of *Helleborus niger* 1000th (B. & T.) he began to pass more urine, until it became profuse, to move occasionally, and very slowly gain consciousness. The first sign that he gave of really comprehending anything was this. He was a boy that had always been particularly fond of money, especially silver money (free silver). While testing him with a lamp one evening to see if I could get his attention to anything, the father said:

"Try him with a piece of money."

I then held a silver dollar in such a position that the lamp would reflect it strongly into his eyes, and for a second he fixed his sight upon it and laugh aloud—"Ha! ha!"

We "ha! ha!'d," too, but it was several days after that before he could see or know enough to indicate what he wanted, or that he wanted anything. He went on improving slowly until perfect recovery under the *Helleborus*. This illustrates the sphere of this remedy anywhere, either in acute meningitis or in typhus, where the affection centers in the head, and with these symptoms.

CLINICAL CASE. ZINCUM METALLICUM.

Zincum metallicum is also a remedy which comes to our help in the last stage of these desperate brain cases. Allow me once more to quote a case from my own work, *Leaders in Homœopathic Therapeutics*, which will show its power here. (See page 145.)

A young lady about twenty years of age complained a week before I was called of weakness, or feeling of general prostration; headache and loss of appetite, but the greatest complaint was of prostration.

She was a student, and her mother, who was an excellent nurse, attributed all her sickness to overwork at school and tried to rest and "nurse her up." But she continued to grow worse. I prescribed for her *Gelsemium*, and followed it with *Bryonia* according to indications, and she ran through a mild course of two weeks longer, and seemed convalescing quite satisfactorily.

Being left in a room alone, while sleeping and perspiring, she threw off the clothes, caught cold and relapsed. Of course the "last state of that patient was worse than the first." The bowels became enormously distended, profuse hemorrhage occurred, which was finally controlled by *Alumen.* A low form of delirium came on, the prostration became extreme notwithstanding the hemorrhage was checked, until the following picture obtained:

Staring eyes rolling upward, head retracted; complete unconsciousness; lying on back and sliding down in bed, twitching, or rather intense, *violent trembling all over*, so that she shook the bed. I had nurses hold her hands night and day, she shook and trembled so; hippocratic face, extremities deathly cold to knees and elbows, pulse so weak and quick I could not count it and intermittent; in short, all signs of impending paralysis of the brain. The case seemed hopeless, but I put ten drops of *Zincum metallicum* 200th (B. & T.) in two drams of cold water and worked one half of it between her set teeth, a little at a time, and an hour after the other half. In about an hour after the second dose she turned her eyes down and faintly said, "*Milk!*" Through a bent tube she swallowed a half glass of milk, the first nourishment she had received in twenty-four hours. She got no more medicine for four days, and improved steadily all the time. She afterwards received a dose of *Nux vomica*, and progressed rapidly to a perfect recovery."

I have now given three remedies that have, *prominently*, *general trembling*, *Gelsemium*, *Apis mellifica* and *Zincum met.* Several others have this symptom, but not so persistently or intensely as these. *Gelsemium* trembling occurs almost wholly in the first week, and the other two in the third or fourth week.

Having now discussed the remedies most generally useful in the different varieties of fever, it remains to notice those other remedies which are exceptionally useful and which in some cases are indispensable. One very important one not mentioned in

Raue, Lilienthal, Johnson or Jahr is

CINA IN TYPHOID.

I once had five cases of typhoid fever in one family, all in bed at the same time. Two took on the most violent form of the cerebral variety, and the other three were of the abdominal type. The youngest, a little girl of about seven years of age, was very sick, having the stupor, unconsciousness, tympany, diarrhœa, dry dark tongue and such other symptoms as generally characterize or make up the diagnosis of abdominal typhus. The ordinary remedies did not seem to do any good. The only thing that the child seemed to notice was a spoon put to her mouth with water, which she would eagerly open her mouth for as often as it touched her lips. There were two other symptoms that were prominent.

Intense *circumscribed redness of the cheeks*, and frequent and *violent rubbing of the nose.*

I hesitated to give *Cina* because this was an undoubted case of typhoid, and no text-book ever said give *Cina.* But I finally gave it, and in the next twenty-four hours my little patient became conscious, and general and rapid improvement set in and continued to perfect recovery.

One evening my telephone rang and a brother physician, in a town sixteen miles away, rehearsed a similar case, asking for advice. I answered "*Cina.*"

"Why, damn it, this is typhoid fever, it isn't worms!" said the doctor.

I answered again, "*Cina*, I don't care what it is."

Two weeks later he came into my office.

"How is that case of worms?" said I.

"Well," said he, "that patient improved from the hour she got the *Cina.* I guess the next time I'll know enough to prescribe according to the symptoms and not for the name of a disease, as you have always taught me."

So it is. The next case of any disease may call for a remedy that no one ever prescribed in that disease, because the symptoms call for it. This is Homœopathy according to Hahnemann's teaching, and the sooner we learn and profit by it the better for us and our patients.

Cina is often neglected because it is generally considered in connection with helminthiasis, not only in fevers, but in rheumatism, where it has aggravation on motion similar to *Bryonia*, and has cured cases where that remedy had failed.

Arnica suffers the same neglect on account of its reputation for effects of bruises, and is given sometimes when *Ledum* or *Sulphuric acid* would be better.

Let us stick to our text, *Similia Similibus Curentur.*

AURUM TRIPHYLLUM IN TYPHOID.

I have met a few cases of typhus in which, during its course, the *mouth would be very red, raw and even bloody. The patients would pick and bore into the raw surfaces, tho' doing so gave great pain, causing them to cry out, but still would keep up the boring.* I lost one case of that kind, because I did not know what could be done with

Arum triphyllum. I took one case of this kind, after it had run between two and three weeks under another physician's care, who was giving *Aconite* tincture because *she had fever*, and I cured it promptly with this remedy. A few hours after the first visit I called again, and the mother of the patient (a young lady) said:

"Doctor, did you give Clara morphine?"

I answered, "No! Why?"

"She fell asleep a few minutes after you put the powder on her tongue, and has been sleeping perfectly natural since, which she has not done for several days and nights past."

These symptoms of the mouth

are oftener found in scarlet fever than in typhoid, but that makes no difference, it is *similia*, etc., just the same and no remedy can be substituted for *Arum triphyllum* here. The fever runs very high in such cases, and a high grade of delirium with such a mouth is no counter indication.

VERATRUM ALBUM, CAMPHORA AND SECALE CORNUTUM IN TYPHOID.

If during the course of a typhoid case there occurs—"*Sudden and rapid sinking of vital force; to complete prostration; cold sweat*, especially upon the face and forehead; *cold breath; face hip-*

pocratic; nose pointed and cold, a picture of general collapse, no remedy can equal *Veratrum album.*

In such a case do not give alcoholic stimulants, for this remedy can do much better. After it has helped us out of this state of collapse, other remedies, according to indications, will generally be needed to conduct the case along to recovery.

Camphor comes the nearest to *Veratrum album* as a remedy for this collapse, of *rapid onset*, (unlike *Carbo vegetabilis* which comes on gradually), but the *Camphor* while cold all over, with sweats, does not so characteristically present the cold *sweat upon the forehead*, and *Camphor* has a very prominent symptom not found under *Veratrum album*, *viz.*, notwithstanding the objective coldness *the patient cannot bear to be covered.* This latter symptom should also call to mind *Secale cornutum* which has the same. Here are three remedies which are liable to be indicated in collapse occurring in typhoid. It may be objected that these are remedies that are generally most useful in Asiatic cholera, when indicated by such symptoms. True, because oftener indicated there than elsewhere, but here let me repeat and *emphasize* that the name of the disease cannot decide the choice of the remedy, but the symptoms must. So if in exceptional cases, even of typhoid, such symptoms should appear, not to prescribe one of these remedies in accordance with our *law of cure* would not only be unscientific, but criminal.

ANTI-PSORIC REMEDIES IN TYPHOID.

There are four anti-psoric remedies that should always be kept in mind when treating a case of typhoid. They are *Sulphur*, *Calcarea ostrearum*, *Lycopodium clavatum* and *Silicea*.

We have already given the leading indications for *Sulphur*.

CALCAREA.

Calcarea ostrearum.—If at, or about, the beginning of the third week of the fever the *exanthem*, or miliary rash, has not made its appearance, and the other symptoms are not being controlled by other remedies, a few doses of *Calcarea ost.* may develop the rash and stop the diarrhœa, if present, and so modify the case that the rest of the course is easily managed. *Calcarea* may be given whether diarrhœa or constipation is present.

LYCOPODIUM.

Lycopodium clavatum has served me well when at or about the same time in the course of the disease there was present—great *meteoristic distension of the abdomen*, with much rumbling. Constipation, delayed exanthem, sopor, and, especially, *when awaking*, *exceedingly cross*, *irritable*, *kicking or jerking the limbs*, *scolding or screaming*. Urine scanty and red, or clear with *red sandy sediment*. Now, if in addition to all this the symptoms are generally worse from four to eight P. M. no remedy can act more beautifully than *Lycopodium clavatum*. I have seen it clean up the whole case, and in very short order, too.

SILICEA.

Silicea.—I have also had occasion to use this remedy in a very obstinate and long running case of this disease, in which the patient was greatly reduced and had very *profuse sweating*. He also wished to be constantly rubbed, or magnetized, and seemed greatly comforted thereby. A few doses of *Silicea* 6m., Jenichen, changed the whole aspect of this discouraging case, and all went well until complete recovery.

HÆMORRHAGES IN TYPHOID.

As regards the hæmorrhages which occur in this disease, I have found most useful the following remedies:

Alumina.—If the discharge of blood occurs in a coagulated mass, resembling liver, with serum, without much pain, but great weakness.

Alumen serves equally well in such cases.

Hamamelis Virginica has acted well when the blood was *very dark*, venous blood, and there was sensation of great soreness in the abdomen. In addition to the internal use of the remedy I have laid cloths wet with the tincture over the abdomen.

Nitric acid.—When the hemorrhages were mostly bright red, not clotted blood, active hemorrhage, and especially if the patient had been subject to anal troubles before the fever.

Arnica montana.—Blood bright red, also, but clotted.

Terebinthina.—If there is with the hemorrhage *extreme tympanitis* and a bright red tongue, *smooth and glossy*, as if deprived of its papillæ.

China officinalis.—If the patient has lost a large amount of blood already, and there is fainting, ringing in the ears, loss of sight and especially if later on or during convalesçence the effects of the loss of blood are long lasting.

After all, it must be remembered that these remedies are only recommended here for this particular feature of a typhoid case, and that hemorrhage is *only a symptom*, and while it may be necessary to interpolate a remedy for it we must place our main dependence upon the generally indicated remedy for the cure of the patient. It will be remembered that in our treatment of the general remedies hæmorrhage occurs under several of them, and they will generally control this symptom with the rest of the case. Indeed, if those remedies are skillfully used it is very seldom that hæmorrhage will ever occur. No one symptom, be it ever so prominent, should engross the attention of the physician, to the degree of leading him away from a close scrutiny of the whole case.

LIVER COMPLICATIONS IN TYPHOID.

We may sometimes get liver complications in a case that is decidedly typhoid in its generality. If in such a case the tongue becomes *thickly coated yellow* with red edges, the stools are very yellow, *yellow as gold;* the urine also very yellow, whites of eyes yellow, and especially if the patient complains of pains in the region of liver, running across the abdomen, or under the right shoulder blade, no good homœopath would hesitate to give *Chelidonium majus.* There is another remedy having a tongue *coated yellow at the base* and, in connection, there is foul smelling breath, with tongue showing imprints of the teeth; it is *Mercurius protojodatus.* It does well here and it is the only preparation of *Mercury* that I have known to do any good in cases of a typhoid nature.

Of course in bilious remittent fever it is different, and *Mercury* may be very useful, but, as a rule, the more typhoid, the less *Mercury*.

A LEPTANDRA VIRGINICA CASE.

Leptandra Virginica once rendered me very good service in a case that I took from another physician, who had so far failed to get very good results from his treatment, and the particular indication leading me to select it was *dark fetid tarry stools*, mixed with blood and mucus. The patient was greatly prostrated and would have died, I think, but for the timely use of this remedy.

A MELILOTUS CASE.

I once had two cases in one family, one of which taking on the pneumonic type was greatly benefited by *Hyoscyamus niger;* the other of the cerebral form had attack after attack of the most profuse epistaxis I ever saw. No remedy seemed in the least to control these attacks until after observing that each attack was preceded by the *most intense redness of the face* I gave *Melilotus officinalis* 30th. This was followed by complete relief, not only of the epistaxis, but a decided amelioration of all the symptoms, and an easily managed case until recovery.

ANTIMONIUM TARTARICUM.

Antimonium tartaricum ought to be mentioned as a very useful remedy in pneumo-typhus, when the lungs or bronchi become so loaded with mucus, that cannot be expectorated, that marked *cyanosis is present*. There is coarse, rattling breathing, and when coughing it seems as if a whole cupful of mucus must come up, but none comes. The patient cannot raise it. Here a few doses of this remedy does wonders by enabling the patient to expectorate, thereby relieving the embarrassed respiration. There may have to be made a choice between this remedy and *Carbo vegetabilis*, *Veratrum album* or *Lycopodium clavatum*.

ALWAYS THE LAW.

Now, after giving the leading indications for so many remedies, we are not forgetful of the truth that there are many other valuable symptoms that may come in to make up the perfect picture, which have not been mentioned. So, after all, it remains for every prescriber to recognize and apply all that is lacking, according to our unerring law of cure. But there must be a *starting* point in every case, and this so far as we are able, is what we have attempted to furnish. Further; not only have we not given *all* the indications, but are also aware that we have not mentioned all the remedies that may possibly come into a case of typhus. In fact, there is no remedy, in or out of our large armamentarium, that may not be indicated in some exceptional case. This is the wide field from which new harvests are yet to be garnered. Where are the reapers? Nevertheless, I am confident that with even our present knowledge in homœopathic therapeutics we are vastly better able to cope successfully with this disease than any other school of medicine.

PREMONITORY SYMPTOMS AND CONVALESCENCE.

I will now call attention to some indications for remedies that I have found useful for the symptoms that threaten an attack; and, also, for the stage of convalescence therefrom.

Every case has its beginnings. They may be so small as to at first escape observation, or may seem so trivial as to need no attention. But, remember, that the day of small things is, after all, often the important time, and that the "stitch in time that saves nine" is a truism that can nowhere be more clearly proven than in the early scientific prescription. I am fully persuaded that many a case of typhoid has been prevented from ever reaching the stage where it could certainly be diagnosed as such, by this kind of prescribing.

So if we find, especially during an epidemic of typhus—"lassitude and heavy limbs with headache, white covered tongue, loss of appetite, belching, or with these gastric symptoms acute shooting pains in different parts of the body, the patient wanting to *lie perfectly still because worse on movement*," a few doses of *Bryonia alba.* will both clear out these *symptoms* and dispel our fears, whether the case was actually typhus incipiens, or not.

If, with suspended catamenia, we have coated tongue with bad, or bitter, taste in the mouth especially in the morning, with bitter or sour belching, *heat unbearable*, *but uncovering makes* her *chilly*, *Pulsatilla* 30th will set all to rights.

If nothing much is complained of but great *weakness or prostration*, can hardly move because *so weak*, and when does move *trembles all over* from weakness, *Gelsemium nitidum* 30th. I have never received more hearty expressions of gratitude for sensible relief than from patients who have experienced the effects of this remedy in such cases.

If, with a feeling of prostration, there is a coated tongue, which is flabby, with a dry red tip, not so distinctly triangular as that of *Rhus toxicodendron*, but approaching it, and a sore, bruised feeling all over, which makes the patient complain of the hardness of everything lain upon, and hard aching pain in head, back, and limbs, there is no remedy like *Baptisia tinctoria*.

I generally give it in the 30th in frequently repeated doses until I get an effect, then stop it or lengthen the intervals between doses.

Belladonna has often relieved when there was severe throbbing congestive headache, < lying down, with drowsiness but inability to sleep, temperature high and pulse quick.

Cocculus in cases that have become worn out with watching, and loss of sleep; all tired out, can hardly hold the head up, *neck feels so weak.* (*Nitric acid.*)

Nux vomica in cases that have been closely confined in-doors by business, persons of sedentary habits, or of intellectual pursuits; who become constipated, stomach gets out of order, food distresses, sleep is unrefreshing, feels worse in the morning than any other time; is a little feverish, with *red face*, *yet wants to be covered*, or in warm room, quiet, as the *least movement* or *uncovering makes him chilly.*

All these states that I have pictured under these different remedies may precede an attack of typhus, which will never fully develop if properly met by the appropriate remedy at the outset. I might add indications for other remedies, but these alone will cover most cases, and every physician must learn to be on the alert for any case that comes outside of them.

This is his *business.*

During the stage of *convalescence* it is scarcely less important that we should be able to prescribe correctly than in the incipiency of an attack of typhus, because many a relapse has, and may, occur without it, and there are affections known as sequelæ of typhus which may be prevented if properly treated.

Psorinum is one of our best remedies if, during convalescence, the patient is *hopeless*, in complete despair of recovery, notwithstanding he is really getting better; the appetite delays, weakness continues, with night sweats, or sweats on the least movement that requires effort. A dose of *Psorinum* 500th helps wonderfully in such cases.

China officinalis is also good for the night sweats, or sweats on the least effort, with great weakness and slow return of strength, especially if during its course the case was attended with a great *loss of blood* or other vital fluids; there may still remain some brownish diarrhœa, or the appetite may be *poor*, or *canine*, and digestion *slowly* performed, with accumulation of gas which bloats the abdomen causing an uncomfortable feeling of *fullness as if the abdomen were packed full.*

In one case of typhus, which was, I think, the worst from which I ever saw a patient recover, after the worst had been passed, the case dragged along still presenting an unnaturally high temperature and pulse, < in A. M., face red, with chilliness on uncovering or moving. *Nux vomica* 200th put in the "finishing touch" and brought on rapid improvement until complete recovery.

Cocculus is also to be studied in cases where, with delayed appetite, a feverish feeling still remains.

Veratrum album, strength alone wanting (Jahr.)

Anacardium orientale, loss of memory.

Ignatia amara, one-sided headaches.

Pulsatilla, appetite too ravenous.

Arnica, *Phosphorus*, or *Petroleum*, deafness remaining.

Sulphur. If the feet burn, or there are occasionally flashes of fever, passing off with moisture, a sense of debility, and to prevent chronic effects of the disease generally.

Calcarea ostrearum, where the patient is of the *Calcarea* temperament, and evidently inclined to tubercular deposit, particularly if there is any cough and soreness in the chest.

As we said when writing of the remedies for the incipient stage, these are only a few of the remedies that may be indicated. We may "watch out" for others that are equally efficacious. There is great satisfaction in finishing up a case well.

THE SICK ROOM AND CARE OF THE PATIENT.

In regard to the sick room, I give my patients all the fresh air I can, without subjecting them to dangerous exposure.

Fresh air is the best disinfectant, and the nurse should wear enough clothing if it is cold weather to protect herself also. This is especially necessary when the fever is running high.

The temperature of the room should be graduated according to the intensity of the fever.

Bathing, especially during the height of the fever, should be frequently performed, and if there is much sweating or disposition thereto, under the clothes. Towels are better than sponges.

Burned coffee is as good as any disinfectant, aside from fresh air.

Carbolic acid, Chloride of Lime, Iodoform, etc., are abominations and more injurious than any odor arising from the patient. Platt's chlorides are better.

The bedding should be changed frequently, being well aired, and the changing performed with as little excitement as possible.

Never interrupt sleep. Stupor is not sleep.

I let my patients have all the cold or warm water they want to drink, unless it causes distress, nausea, or vomiting. Never give melted ice, but water cooled by ice around the outside of the vessel containing it. Dried apple water is a beautiful beverage. It is refreshing, nutritious, and acts gently upon the kidneys, increasing the urine.

For the regular nourishment I have for twenty-five years used *oat meal gruel* when I could get my patients to take it. I let them have it warm or cold, as they desire, and encourage them to take it freely. I do not know anything better.

I prepare it as follows: Put a large handful into a pint of cold water, let it stand an hour or two, then set it on the stove and cook it until it is all soft, keeping the dish full of water. Then strain out the coarse part through a cloth, take the liquid portion, and while it is hot add an equal quantity of fresh sweet milk, salt to taste. Most patients like it at the outset, and those who do not will often become very fond of it after taking it a few times. But once in a great while a patient will not like it. Then milk with rice, prepared the same way, or wheat flour and milk, come next. But of course the diet question cannot be absolutely settled alike for all patients.

Alcoholic stimulants are no good. Proper food with the homœopathic remedy is all that is needed.

Care must be taken, when returning to the ordinary mixed diet, not to overload; and, at the same time, to give enough of kind and quality to sustain and nourish. One of the greatest dangers is in gratifying to repletion an abnormal craving, though I have found, on the other hand, that if the patient greatly desired any particular article, and could not be satisfied without it, that it was best to give it, but very carefully. I learned this from a curious experience. I had a fever patient who, during the height of her fever, was continually calling piteously for lemons. This was in my earlier practice. She continued to grow worse, notwithstanding my best efforts, for I had been taught that lemons would *antidote* certain remedies and thought that she could not bear a raw lemon on her stomach at this time any way. Finally my old preceptor, Dr. T. L. Brown, was called in consultation. The moment he came into the room she exclaimed:

"Oh, Dr. Brown, can't I have a lemon?"

He looked at her a moment, then said: "Do you want a *lemon?*"

"Oh! yes!"

"Give her a lemon." One was handed her, and we sat looking at her until in about one minute that whole lemon, except rind and seeds, was swallowed. That woman improved from that moment and never called for another in her life, that I know of.

I have seen a patient devour a medium-sized cucumber pickle the same way. Dr. Santee, just in my office, says he allowed a patient to eat a half dozen raw oysters with vinegar, which she very much desired, and with great satisfaction and benefit, notwithstanding an allopathic doctor who had a typhoid patient in the same house said she would die. While this is true, and convalescence may be retarded by denying the patient what she so greatly craves, yet such cravings must be carefully relieved for over-doing will be disastrous, as I have also had occasion to witness.

Another danger is in allowing the patient to get up and around too soon. "Make haste slowly" is here the best maxim and should be faithfully heeded. Over-exertion of mind or body is very presumptuous. Abstain from too early sexual intercourse. It has proved fatal.

So far as artificial foods are concerned, I have not used them much. Where digestion continued weak I have occasionally used Mellin's Food, giving a teacupful prepared according to their formula, after meals. It has seemed to me not only to furnish aliment in itself, but to aid the digestion of the food taken before it.

Hoping this little book may aid my brethren, especially the younger men in our ranks, I now close.

INDEX.

A

B

C

D

E

F

G

H

I

K

L

P

R

S